Being in a Body

By
Rev. Victoria Pendragon, D.D.

For permission, serialization, condensation, adaptions, or for our catalog of other publications, write to Ozark Mountain Publishing, Inc., P.O. Box 754, Huntsville, AR 72740, ATTN: Permissions Department.

Library of Congress Cataloging-in-Publication Data

Victoria Pendragon – 1946-

Being in a Body by Victoria Pendragon

Being in a Body is a kind of an "owner's guide" to your body except for the fact that we don't actually "own" our bodies; we're just along for the ride... so perhaps it's a bit more like driving instructions for the elegant and finely tuned vehicle the human body is.

1.Healing 2. Consciousness 3.Self Help 4. Metaphysical
I. Pendragon, Victoria 1946 II. Metaphysical III. Consciousness IV. Title

Library of Congress Catalog Card Number: 2020940674
ISBN: 9781940265834

Cover Art and Layout: Victoria Cooper Art
Book set in: Litania, Times New Roman, Litania
Book Design: Summer Garr
Published by:

OZARK
MOUNTAIN
PUBLISHING

PO Box 754, Huntsville, AR 72740
800-935-0045 or 479-738-2348; fax 479-738-2448
WWW.OZARKMT.COM

Printed in the United States of America

Content

"There is a form of Japanese art called Kintsugi, which dates back to the 15th century. In it, masters repair broken plates and cups and bowls, but instead of simply fixing them back to their original state, they make them better. The broken pieces are not glued together, but instead fused with a special lacquer mixed with gold or silver."

—Ryan Holiday, *How to Recover when the World Breaks You*, 2018

This book is dedicated to my body, a remarkable body that has survived two "fatal," "incurable" diseases, one of which—diffuse progressive systemic sclerosis— turned her skin, muscles, tendons, and much of her internal organs into scar tissue. She is also a body that endured a remarkable amount of sexual abuse when she was very young, abuse that led to an expansion of "my" consciousness of how the world and energy work. Her wise guidance saved both my life and my mind and opened me up to numerous extra-physical gifts.

I am Kintsugi.

My name is Victoria Pendragon and this book is about what I have learned about being in a body as the result of being broken and put back together again. My conscious healing process has unfolded over a period of about thirty-six years so far. I imagine that it will most likely continue for the remainder of my life as each step that I take toward being clear of my past seems to allow me deeper access to smaller wounds that had not been so obvious at first.

I have made a commitment to my body to heal. She deserves it.

I am the author of, among other things, three self-help books on do-it-yourself emotional cellular reprogramming. The technique that I teach was gifted to me in 2003 by a disembodied voice that came to me as I slept, woke me up, and stayed with me until it had gotten its point across. I was, at that time, sixteen years into a career as a shamanic healer, a career that I had also been "gifted with" as a result of surviving two fatal and incurable diseases, one that remade my body from head to foot, inside and out. My body is a kind of a miracle and, I suppose, a rare creature. She has done the unlikely twice, having also healed from an illness that should also have proved fatal when she was six months old. I am an artist and a scribe for her, doing my best to bring you the information that I have been privileged to have been given access to.

Every human being is a kind of a miracle because

1

each of us is far more than most people have been led to believe. Each of us is a three-part entity. At some level of consciousness, humanity has always known this because, if you look back in time, you will find that at least two of the world's currently existing largest religions espouse a three-part God. Christianity goes with the construct of a Father, Son, and Holy Ghost, while Hinduism goes for the Trimurti, which consists of Brahma, Vishnu, and Shiva. I like to think that way back before these religions first came into being, in times that were more firmly rooted in the need to survive, the mystics of older, supposedly more primitive religions may have, at some level, tapped into the fact that we, ourselves—human beings—are, in fact, three-part beings, and that the gods that have been created over the centuries are refined versions of their own existence.

Ed Stafford, an extreme survivalist, in his book, *Under the Skin,* tells of aboriginal wisdom:

"The Aboriginals teach that the body has three brains: The gut, the heart, and the head. Instinct lives in the gut, the belly. They caution that one must rely on the brain in the belly because the instinct will always know best. Their name for the brain in the head is nan-du-ka-ru which, loosely translated, refers to a tangled fishing net, essentially a mess that one cannot get out of."

In the seventeenth century, Rene Descartes, who was to break ground in the fields of both philosophy and mathematics, also posited the existence of humans as three-parted beings, partially because of the importance of dreams in his life. The list of creative individuals, military and political figures, scientists and inventors who have brought lasting changes to the ways that we live and think is long, and many of these individuals "brought forth" these ideas from dreams, using their very good minds to translate images, ideas, and visions from an invisible realm in ways that could be shared with others, moving humanity along its evolutionary path by use of information that was, in every sense, from what might be called an invisible realm: the unconscious mental field.

In about 1986, shortly before my body was to manifest the first symptoms of the usually fatal and incurable disease that is technically known as progressive systemic sclerosis, in every dream that I recalled, I existed as a three-part being. One aspect of me was the leader of the group of three, generally in charge of whatever was going on. Another aspect of me was always—always!—dead asleep and had to be carried everywhere by the third aspect of me, who seemed to exist solely for the purpose of carrying around the sleeping version of me, who was out cold.

I didn't know what to make of the dreams at the time but I sensed strongly that they were trying to tell me something … I just didn't know what.

By the time the early nineties rolled around and the doctors had declared my body and blood to be entirely free of the disease I'd had, those dreams had vanished. I can't tell you exactly when they stopped but it was at some point during those years when my life was dedicated solely to the healing of my body. In retrospect, I suspect that my mind—let's call that aspect of myself Victoria #1—was the leader of that dream group, setting the goals for the group and leading it wherever it wanted to go, ignorant of the struggles that Victoria #2, who was carrying around Victoria #3, was experiencing. I suspect that Victoria #2 represented my poor, beleaguered body which had been pressed into service carrying my Spirit Self aspect—Victoria #3—through every poor decision and experience that Victoria #1—who represented my mind—had involved them in.

"Rather than *mind* and *our own will*, studies in Biology and Genetics have shown the body is more of an authority—and a better indicator—on who and what we are.

Additionally, neuroscientific research using brain scans has shown that decisions are made seven seconds before we are even aware of the need to make a decision—confirming that the mind is not in control of our decision making.

The last several decades have seen advances in our understanding of the body, the brain, and the nature of consciousness. Those advances have brought clarity to the mystery of who we are and how we operate." (Jovian Archives, 2019)

The Mind

Let's start exploring this internal hierarchy that I imagine with the troublemaker, since it's the one-third of the threesome that in most people has been put in charge by default both because of the tremendous emphasis that is placed on it and because of all the input it receives throughout childhood: The mind.

Most parents put the Mind on a throne … And there, for most people, it tends to stay throughout their lives. The information that all of us receive in childhood provides the foundation for how we learn to live our lives. It also provides the foundation for what we learn to expect from life. This happens because our bodies both take in and hold on to everything that they come in contact with via their senses. The more feeling energy or emotional energy there is around the information that comes into the body, the more firmly anchored that information becomes. We are quite literally programmed by the people who raise us.

It only takes seven years to firmly anchor information in the body and, since the body of a child is an almost clean slate, the first information that it takes in from the outside world easily finds a foothold. A child growing inside its mother's uterus is also being programmed. The timing of a complete turnover of the cells of the body—seven years—has been scientifically proven but it was known about long before. It is said that the Jesuits had an old saying, "Give me a child until he is seven years old and he is mine for life." So this information has been well known for centuries. Now, we know why.

The Mind is generated by our very physical human brain. It is, metaphorically, the child born of the Body and the Spirit Self, and like a child born of human parents, it can mitigate between the two when they are at odds, acting in the role of go-between. I will, from this point on, be referring to this ineffable vitalizing factor of the human being as the "Spirit Self" in order to distinguish it both from the broader term "spirit," referring to the larger overarching spirit of the universe, as well as to distinguish it from the other intangible associated with the body: the Mind. The Mind knows what the Body knows because all of the cells of the body carry all of the information of a person's lifetime and, as the cells reproduce, cells of the body pass that information on to the new generation. As new cells come into being to replace dying cells, they receive the history of that human being as part of who they are. The human *body* never forgets anything; the information may degrade a little as years pass by, but the *feeling* essence of the information is always there. Techniques like emotional cellular reprogramming and SleepMagic—which is emotional cellular reprogramming that you do yourself—can do what I call de-fusing the emotional component of a cellular memory, which is helpful for the person carrying that memory if the memory is traumatic or disturbing in any way, but the core memory itself—the cellular knowledge of what happened—remains.

The brain—which is physical—is made up of cells, just like the rest of the body's cells, and those brain cells also carry the information that the rest of the body carries. But the energy that the brain generates—the mind, as we call it—is one step *removed* from the physicality of the body in that the mind is *not* physical and therefore does not have a cellular structure. This is what makes it possible for the Mind to be a kind of a go-between, mitigating ongoing transmissions between the physical body and the information that it carries in its cells and the ephemeral information generated by the Spirit Self.

It's not a perfect system.

If you've ever been in a situation that required a translator, attempting to have a conversation or acquire some information from someone who spoke a language with which you had no familiarity, or if you've spoken with someone who is new to your language and does not have a grasp on some of the subtle differences that exist in your language, nor do you have any grasp of the subtleties of theirs, then you can imagine the sorts of problems that might exist for the offspring mind of the physical body attempting to translate from spirit to body or from body to spirit. The Mind is a little of both but not entirely either so the best it can do, without training, is to make do.

Translation from spirit to body is a lot more like a warm-blooded animal attempting communication with a cold-blooded animal than it is like translating from one language to another, or even between one member of the warm-blooded species to another. While you may have heard of horse whisperers or dog whisperers it's less likely that you've heard of, for instance, a cricket whisperer. Not that it couldn't happen; anything can happen; but it would certainly be a rare occurrence.

I am Kintsugi.

So here we are, Beings in Bodies with a go-between for communicating with each other—the Mind—that has acquired that job because, generally speaking, that's what we've been taught to do: use our minds. Minds are excellent for making hard, physical calculations—math, science, etc. But when it comes around to "figuring out" things like the ineffable subtleties of emotion, the mind struggles. You can pin down numbers and elements but it's difficult to sort out the subtle quirks and twists of emotional responses. We have learned to live with that because we have been *taught* to live with that when, in fact, we have at our disposal something built into us that is much more facile at dealing with emotions: the voice of the body, a voice children are rarely taught to listen for despite the fact that the phrase "listen to your gut" is something we often hear once we have moved into a more mature state and have, by that time, been distanced from it.

By that time, most of us have come to rely so heavily on the Mind that our tendency is to "interpret" our gut feelings and responses, not *listen* to them. There's a big difference.

We are made up of a spiritual element that has combined with a physical element and we have been taught to utilize our physically generated minds to get us through life when our bodies actually carry far more intelligence—intrinsic intelligence—that we can work with to make a life that can more perfectly reflect the Spirit Self that came to Earth to learn and grow and discover by way of existing in a physical, animal form.

Once we master our own challenge, we can move on to discover how to be in a physical being that is in relationship to *other* Spirit Selves inhabiting other physical beings. The first relationship we have to learn to handle, though, is the most critically important relationship in our lives as humans: the relationship between our Spirit

7

Self and our body and the role of the mind *inside* of that relationship. In other words, we will best handle relationships with others, once we learn how to handle our own integral relationship of Body, Mind, and Spirit Self.

Perhaps the best place to start learning to navigate yourself is to begin to grow accustomed to thinking of yourself as the three-part being that you are. This is precisely the sort of discipline that your mind exists to handle. It is the mind that "thinks" but what the mind thinks is very dependent upon what has been "fed" *to* the mind. That particular "brain food" comes from many sources. It can come from the body itself and from the feelings that the body generates, some of which are energetic and emotional, while others are purely physical. Other brain food comes from outside sources—other people, for instance, and various kinds of media, as well as from life experiences.

Information that we receive when we are very young—even when we are in utero—is often information that is repeated since we are surrounded, as infants and children, with a relatively small group of people whose energetic information (both emotional and electromagnetic) and whose transmitted verbal information we are exposed to on a regular basis. This exposure, besides influencing our thinking, also energetically conditions us to the acceptance—or rejection—of that thinking and the extrapolations of that thinking.

Tribalism, for instance, is both a part of our physical DNA and of our social DNA. If we grow up with a group of people that are tribally oriented, it is most likely that we, too, will be tribally oriented unless something that is capable of overriding that conditioning happens to us or around us. What we think and the way we think begins before we are even aware that we *can* think.

Generally, throughout most of humankind's

existence on Earth, children have been taught *what* to think, not *how* to think. When the concept of philosophy—essentially the teaching of thinking—ultimately appeared, arising from humankind observing the thinking process objectively, people became more aware of different ways of thinking, but it was not until the twentieth century that anyone began to think about *children* thinking ... and, of course, children *do* think. Not only that, but, as it turns out, the thinking that children do affects everything about the way that they come to view the world and ultimately enter into the activities of the world.

Not until very recently has anyone given any thought to teaching children the many ways in which they can use their minds. Most children are expected to "absorb" from their environment what they need to survive in that particular home. They are "told what to do." Rarely are children taught how to *use* their minds. School is supposed to take care of that but for the most part schools do pretty much the same thing that parents do, they tell children what to do and they tell them whatever version they have learned of how the world is. Generally, there is very little opportunity in school—for young children at any rate—for creative interaction from a thinking standpoint. For that matter, if we were to take the whole world into account, very few teenagers or adults have ever been taught—literally, taught—how to make the best use of their minds. Certainly, the vast majority of people are never taught about the intelligence of their bodies and how to best make use of that.

And now, for a bit of backstory.

Backstory

Before I became ordained, and before I studied to become an honorary Doctor of Divinity, I was both writer and artist. My writings were first published in a national magazine when I was a senior in high school. I wanted to go to college and study journalism. My mother had other ideas.

My mother, when she was very young, had been "pushed" through elementary school and high school by her ambitious father because he saw her remarkable intelligence and, having made and lost his fortune by the time she was in school, had determined that all of his children would become doctors so that they would never find themselves destitute, and the sooner they became doctors, the better because he needed the money. He needed to ensure that when he grew old someone would be able to support him. So, while my mother wanted to become a librarian, she found herself instead as the youngest woman to have entered medical school in the United States at that time.

I guess, that because she had experienced being forced to follow a path that had been set by her father, she felt entitled to set my path as well. Thus it was that, despite my early publication and promise, I ended up in art school. I had no idea what I wanted to do there. I liked art well enough; I always had. But my mother "saw something in me." Thus it was that I graduated college with a BFA and went to work selling ladies shoes. I was unsatisfied and unhappy so I married the first man who asked me—he seemed nice enough—and I discovered that I was still unsatisfied and unhappy.

I have not, thus far, explained much about my childhood, but at this point, by way of explanation, it becomes relevant because my childhood made me a poor candidate both for marriage and for being a mother. I am, at this point in my life (in my seventies as I write this), utterly bored with the story of my life but it needs to be summed up here so that you can see how it was that I came to know everything that I know now about being in a body.

I am Kintsugi.

Summation: at six months of age I "catch" tuberculosis from my mother, who picked it up in the autopsy room at the hospital where she worked. There was no cure for tuberculosis at that time so my mother was sent to the tropics to rest and, as at that time infants generally died from tuberculosis, I was put into the care of a research project where I lived in an incubator for I don't really know how long. The drugs that they were testing on me apparently worked. Once recovered, I was then put into the care of my mother's parents as she was still recovering, taking in the sun and the air, relaxing in a foreign country.

My mother had married a man from the tropics, a Cuban. Her father, an avowed racist, only allowed her to marry the man—also a doctor—because his family was the wealthiest family in Cuba. My grandfather's main concern was always money. He was willing to swap his prejudice for potential security.

Even as an infant, I looked far more like my father than I did like my mother. My skin was a rich olive color, my hair and eyes, deepest brown. Her parents took good care of me though—probably because he had plans for a young brown-skinned girl—and, starting when I was perhaps four or five years old, he put those plans into action, marketing my little body to make money so that he could continue in the lifestyle to which he was accustomed.

Meanwhile, in order to escape from what was happening to me at four or five years old when the abuse began, I began to leave my body. More correctly put, I suppose, my conscious awareness left my body and, for reasons that I still do not know to this day, I would experience myself diving into the Earth as though it were water, swimming through it to find tree roots, which I would then enter into in order to swim up into a tree so that I could watch what was going on below. I could see what was happening to my body and I had some sense of it. Despite the fact that my consciousness was not within my body, I was able to communicate with her—my body—from my safe place in the trees. The trees—wise beings that they are—taught me how to feel what was happening in the bodies of the men who were using my body. The trees taught me how to feel what was happening in the men's bodies so that I could more quickly dispatch them, and get them off of me. That shamanic training—learning how to feel energy moving in others—would, many decades later, help me to help other people heal.

Life at home, with my father and mother, was equally disturbing although that didn't begin until I was seven or eight years old when my father took a liking to me and decided to teach me how to make him happy. My mother knew about it; they had made a deal that his activities would cease when I got my period, for obvious reasons. But it didn't. And there were ramifications.

This highly sexualized childhood and youth created me as a highly sexualized young woman. I was, it seemed to me, physically unable to refuse sex. I wanted to. I hated myself for doing what I did—but I did it all the time. Marriage did literally nothing to change that aspect of who I was. In addition, I'd never really had the benefit of *feeling* loved. My first child seemed to sense my complete inability to love and became what some people might call "a difficult baby." Nothing could satisfy him. Determined to get at least something right, and also to give him someone more his size that he could play with and maybe relate to, I became pregnant again but I went about the process very differently, learning everything I could about how to ensure a good delivery and how to establish a bond with my infant. That worked at least a little because my second child was an angel to be with and, for the first time in my life, I experienced love.

There was a problem, though, as when I had agreed

to marry their father I had told him that I did not want children. I had spent my life as the oldest of eleven and I'd had my fill of taking care of babies. However, once I became aware that I seemed to be completely unable to turn off the promiscuity that I had been so used to, it occurred to me that having a child could make it impossible to behave the way I had been behaving because I simply wouldn't have time or availability to do that. I never told my husband that I had stopped taking birth control pills and he was not happy with my pregnancy.

In retrospect, it's easy to see that my children's father had wanted me to love him, but because we attract to us that which we carry within us, he didn't know how to love me either. Children only made the situation worse and when I became pregnant a third time, he insisted angrily that I have an abortion. I was heartbroken but guilty as well, so I did as I was told, just as I had spent my whole early life doing.

Ultimately, there was a divorce and I lost my children to him as he had threatened to tell them "the kind of person that I was." If I hated me and who I was, I figured, surely my children would hate me too, if they knew who I really was. Less than four years after the divorce, for the second time in my life, I acquired a disease for which there was no cure.

It was that disease—a rapidly advancing case of diffuse progressive systemic sclerosis that turned my body, inside and out, into scar tissue—that brought me to a place from which I would ultimately discover—and grow to appreciate—how magical life can be because what happened to my body as the result of scleroderma (*short form for the previously named disease*) changed everything about what I understood life was and began opening me to the remarkable intelligence of my body and the ever-present spirit being that had determined to come here and live this life.

Scleroderma is a hideously painful disease. The pain is unrelenting and, because there is no known cure for it, there is no real opportunity for hope to put down roots. I had been suffering from it for about a year and a half, unable to find even the slightest relief from the pain and I would spend my nights, as I lay sleepless, auditioning various ways to kill myself. I was frustrated because I could not come up with anything that was foolproof, with anything that might not leave me in possibly even worse shape than I already was.

The body, remember, is filled with information. When that information is emotionally charged it carries energy and when that energy is not dispersed, when it cannot find an outlet, when it is held within the cells of the body which were not designed to hold that particular energy, it can—and often does—cause problems.

The body is filled with useful information. The body knows things that the consciousness may not have access to, as it did in my case. My body held all the knowledge about the abuse she had endured inside the cells of her body which eventually simply couldn't take anymore and broke down, producing, in my case, diffuse progressive systemic sclerosis, a disease so dreadful and so horrifyingly painful that I didn't feel that I could wait for death to come; I just couldn't take any more pain. So my very good mind set about attempting to figure out how it was that I could end my life in a way that was guaranteed to actually *end* my life and not have me end up even worse off than I already was. The result of that was that I discovered—though I didn't understand it at the time—that my body knew way more about what she could do than I did.

Sleep, at the time, was hard to come by unless I was exhausted; the pain kept me awake; any movement I made would send stabbing pains through me, so I lay as still as I could for as long as I could and while I could keep my body still, I had a difficult time keeping my mind still and the subject that my mind was most interested in was how I could commit suicide effectively. One of those many nights I lay awake attempting to figure out how to kill myself, I actually did figure it out. I was thrilled. I was so thrilled that I fell asleep almost immediately.

When I awoke in the morning I remembered briefly having solved my problem, but before my mind could get to work on recalling the details, I found myself literally jumping out of the bed—which should have been impossible as I could barely move at the time since my arms and legs were rigid. Nevertheless, there I was, standing beside the bed with my arms thrown up to the ceiling—which also should have been impossible—saying out loud, at the top of my voice, "Make me an open channel."

The next thing I knew, I was fully awake … unless I had actually been awake when that happened. I didn't know. I was confused. I lay down in bed and closed my eyes and an image appeared in my mind: I saw a hillside, looking mostly like dried grass, only there were seven greenish small bushes growing, four on the bottom row and three on the top. Underneath the bushes were scrawled in a sloppy kind of print, the words, "seven reasons to live."

I had no idea what was going on but I went immediately to the cellar, where my paints were, jammed a paintbrush and some foam into the U-shape that my fingers had taken by then, and painted a small picture of what I had seen. Interestingly, years later, a young neighbor of ours, a teenaged girl who had only recently come out as gay, came into our townhouse to see my paintings, saw that one and commented that it was painted in the exact colors of her bedroom. I knew from having spoken to her earlier that she had been seriously depressed and it seemed to me that those words, "seven reasons to live," in addition to the colors, might have subconsciously drawn her to that work so I gave her the piece. I had healed by then; I'd gotten the message; it seemed like the perfect piece for her and she was very happy to receive it.

That action—my body leaping out of bed when I could barely walk, throwing her arms up to the air, and shouting aloud—that action was all my body's doing. I did not have one conscious thought in my head. That was my body trying to get my attention through her actions and the vision that she had my brain generate, complete with a message for me, a message that made sense in that it clearly stated that I had a reason to live, but it was a message that made no sense to me at the time in saying that I had seven reasons to live.

During the time period that I was working on this manuscript, one early spring morning just at dawn as I was enjoying my daily meditative yoga, standing in—of all things—tree pose, I noticed the scraggly green bushes on the hill, growing up out of fall's dried beige leaves and the dead grasses of winter and I "saw" what I had seen the day I sprang so unexpectedly from bed: seven reasons— and more!—to live.

Time is not linear; it is a continuum and sometimes, some people have access to what they call "the future," which is no future at all, just something that exists at another point on the time continuum. Somehow, it would seem that my body ... or my Spirit Self ... or both ... got access to that and, perhaps determined to stay alive, made sure my mind did too.

Bodies have their secrets.

For reasons I may never know, the consciousness of my body decided to take over on the morning after my Mind had decided how I could end my life. My body's passion for life was so vibrant that she—perhaps fueled by my Spirit Self—took over control, literally jumping me up and off the mattress that was lying on the floor,

I am Kintsugi.

when, on a normal day, she could barely move. My mind had clearly stepped aside.

The Body

The body and the way the body operates provide each of us with a built-in example of how to be in life. When we eat correctly and are able to eat what we require and enough of what we require to keep us healthy and strong, the body functions well. The body can be in energetic integrity because it has been nourished with energetic integrity, with foods that life has designed to work with the bodies that consume it. Different types of bodies need different types of foods.

If a person eats too much, their body lets them know almost immediately that they have eaten too much. A person who is in tune with their body can feel the body shift gears in the exact moment when it has had enough. Even a person who is not in tune with their body will eventually feel the discomfort of having eaten too much. And if that person does not learn from their body over time which foods are the most helpful to eat and how much they should eat, and they continue eating too much on a regular basis, that person will do damage to their body, their health, and their overall well-being.

To be in energetic physical integrity, one has only to do what one *needs* to do, what one is here to do. Each person's body is a perfect example of that. The body—like all animal bodies—does what needs to be done to keep it alive and safe. Thus it is that any decision affecting your life is ideally run past your body's intelligence well before the mind gets involved. The body knows what serves its

survival in the world; the mind knows how to calculate
... and it can also function as a very useful and effective
administrative assistant when there are "rules" to be
followed. The mind excels at rules and the best rules are
the rules that are made up by the body, by observing what
the body responds well to and what it does not respond
well to. The mind, in other words, needs a boss, and that
boss is the body.

Once a body has trained its resident consciousness
to hear its subtle voice, the body's response can be detected
well in advance of actually eating a certain food, drinking
a certain liquid, or performing certain activities. A well-
trained mind will then ensure that a person acts—or does
not act—on the information that it receives from the body.

To be in integrity, ideally everyone would eat
only the foods that resonated correctly with their bodies.
Regrettably, just as most humans are taught the importance
of the function of "the mind," most children are also
taught what they "*need* to eat." Studies were done as long
ago as the 1950s that demonstrated without question that
infants, given a healthy selection of foods to eat, would
perfectly nourish themselves if allowed to pick from an
assortment of healthy foods that were presented to them.
Even at that early stage their bodies knew what to eat.
And, yes, some children would refuse to eat sometimes
... and nothing bad happened. They didn't lose weight
just because from time to time, they might skip a meal.
It's entirely conceivable that the bodies of those children
who chose not to eat at a given mealtime were making
some essential adjustments and simply needed an empty
digestive tract for their bodies to do that work.

Because most people are not allowed, as children,
to exercise that kind of discretion in their meals, a great
many people end up with weight problems and eating
disorders.

The problem was exacerbated by something that

many of you might remember: "the Food Pyramid," which was an illustration of foods that were "required" to "maintain health." The Food Pyramid was originally presented to the general public as a guide to eating correctly, to embrace eating what has come to be known as "a balanced diet." Such guides were first developed early in the twentieth century and, in point of fact, were—and still are—based on ensuring general consumption of the foods that are mass-produced and mass-farmed across the country. In other words, "the Food Pyramid" is and always was more about strengthening the economy than it was about sustaining personal health.

It has finally been more widely accepted that certain types of people cannot eat certain types of food. In many cases, that intolerance is a genetic trait. Things like celiac disease and lactose intolerance are well known to appear in a familial fashion. I first began having difficulty with my digestive tract when I was quite young. My father, before I had reached my twenties and had already endured my first complete upper G.I. series, suggested that I might be lactose intolerant, as he had discovered that he was. As a super fan of cheese and ice cream, I ignored that suggestion and went on eating as I always had. Two decades later I came to discover that my father had been correct.

I had been hospitalized for a major surgery in my thirties and on the day I checked out of the hospital I was feeling remarkably wonderful, feeling far better than I would have expected to feel two days after major surgery. Out of curiosity, I reviewed the foods that I had been given in the hospital and it was the foods that I had *not* been given that stood out: milk and cheese.

I am, by nature—as many people are—reluctant to change, but when undeniable information is presented, I can be moved. I adopted a lactose intolerant approach to eating. My digestive tract improved but it never functioned really wonderfully; it never worked with complete ease and effortlessness until I was in my sixties and discovered, again by chance, that if I refrained from eating grain and a lot of white starchy vegetables, my digestive tract would work effortlessly. Still later, as I moved into my seventies, I discovered that what my body really likes best is to eat simple, whole foods, ideally prepared—simply prepared.

My body doesn't know anything about all these much-touted diets that are around, it just knows how it works and what serves it the best. The same food—and definitely the same diet—simply doesn't work for everyone. It is *your* body that will always know best about what will work for *you*. If you can establish with your body a trusting and deep relationship, your body will share what it knows with you if you train yourself to be open to its messages. Being open to the messages of the body works differently for different people.

One good way to get started in a relationship with your body is to learn about it from an energetic/genetic standpoint and the best ways I know to do that is via Human Design. A PHS (Personal Health System) reading from a trained Human Design analyst can show you how you and the body in which you reside "work." In other words, the reading can show you how to get access to the information that you need to keep your body healthy and operating successfully in life as the person that you came here to be, as the embodied spirit that you are. Also available now are DNA testing kits that can be useful for determining the kind of diet that can work best for your genotype.

Not every body works the same way; there are different energetic types for one thing, and different minds work in different ways as well, which is only logical since they are generated by different types of bodies. It is of tremendous value to know how you, as the individual being that you are, work, because if the information that you are basing how you live your life and how you feed your body is information that came from someone who works differently than you do, then it's very apt to be incorrect information for you and your body.

That said, there are also many things that bodies have intrinsically in common. For example, if you cut them, they bleed; they require oxygen to breathe; they all require fuel of some sort and food is that fuel. Bodies respond to energy. That is one of the things that bodies do best. The fact that bodies respond to energy is what lies behind people "getting a feeling about" something. That "feeling" is the body's response to energy. This is useful in thousands of different ways every day and has literally saved the lives of countless people. Because the body responds to energy, it can be thrown off in its performance of certain everyday tasks—like digesting food—by being in the presence of energy that does not feel good to it. Some people, like myself, have to ensure, if they want to digest their food properly, that they eat in a place that is relatively calm. Apparently, if the energy level in a place is too high, my particular body reads it as potentially dangerous to some degree, focuses its energy on being alert instead of on digesting food, and the end result is a less-than-desirable situation both for my body and myself.

The body responding to energy is also why it is capable of healing via the various modalities of healing that utilize energy. Reiki may be the most well-known of energetic healing modalities but there are countless others and each individual shaman has their own way of running energy. Every person carries this healing energy and, for the most part, what training or initiations do is to introduce people in ways to act properly with others when performing healing. The training also helps people to have confidence in the fact that they really can run energy. This is another thing that most people are not taught in childhood, though even as children, everyone can run energy. (That's why I wrote the book, *Born Healers*; because every one of us can run energy; we are, as the song says, born that way.)

One way that you can prove this to yourself, should you want to, is a very simple technique that works wonderfully well. I will first tell you a little story about an accident I had in which I utilized the technique and, despite the fact that I'd already made use of it in numerous ways, and knew that it worked, I was really quite amazed by the results.

Here's how I found out exactly how well this technique works:

I had spent the day in downtown Philadelphia, shopping, hoping to pick up some useful items for my Feng Shui clients. It had been a long day and it was growing dark when I returned later than I'd expected to return. I had a class scheduled for that evening at my house. A number of the things that I had purchased were rather fragile and I was careful in carrying them up the three tall-ish cement stairs that led to my front door. It could be that I was paying more attention to being careful than I was paying to the stairs I was ascending. I tripped. I remained fully conscious that the items that I was carrying were breakable in the extreme and had been somewhat expensive as well. I put their well-being in front of my own and held them out and away from my body as I crashed to the stairs.

The weather was warm, my legs were bare, as were my arms. My limbs contacted the cement stairs with force as I attempted to save my treasures. I arose carefully and could see that I had been successful in saving my treasures; I, however, was a mess, with bloody shins and forearms. I thought to myself quietly, "that's gonna bruise." Then I remembered the technique that I had learned and used countless times for many minor injuries, usually simply to ensure that I would not have pain or a black and blue mark. I had not applied the technique to any injury quite as serious as the ones I had just received but I figured that, unlike the injuries themselves, it couldn't hurt to try, so I did.

Not only did it work, but I did not, in fact, bruise at all, nor did I experience any pain after the fact. I was amazed. I promise that you can be as well, so here goes: let's say that you have used your forearms to break a fall; you have arisen unbloodied but can tell from the pain you are experiencing that your body is likely to show your injuries boldly. Get yourself up off the ground if that is possible (and, if not, you can perform the operation in a lying or sitting position) and locate a spot above the injury—which is to say, a spot that is higher up your arm and closer to your shoulder—(energy proceeds from the trunk, at about heart level, outward) and then lightly, with your right hand just hovering over your left arm, imagine that you are capturing, in the palm of that right hand, the energy that flows from your torso out and down your arm. Now, without touching the injured arm, as if there were a small force field between your hand and the arm, draw your hand from the shoulder area, down the arm, over the injured area, and out through the hand on that side.

Do that three times.

You can then use the left hand to do the same on the right arm.

That's it. It works like a miracle to mitigate pain and jumpstart healing. You are assisting your body in healing itself. You are caring for a body that you have carelessly injured, letting your body know that you care and, not only that you care, but that you are competent as well, that you can help him or her or them to recover from your own lack of attention.

It works on any part of the body for simple surface injuries.

Please notice that I used the phrase "him or her or them" when referring to your body. My body is "she." Nobody's body is an "it." When I speak to my body I address her as "you" because she is a living being charged with serious and challenging tasks that I seem to bring her on a regular basis. I respect and appreciate her and I speak to her—and with her—in a way that shows respect.

It's easy enough to speak *to* your body but, if you have been used to relying on your mind for feedback and/ or decision making, it may take you a while to be able to really converse with or "hear" what your body is saying to you. That's because the body's language is feeling and sensing. And, if you have gone through life treating your body the way that many people do—as though he or she or they are there simply to carry out your wishes and desires—it may take you a bit longer to communicate effectively than it might if you were simply dealing with another person.

I hope that the following story will illustrate this kind of communication for you and what is possible with this type of communication.

A SleepMagic Story, August 2018

That morning, all I could remember was that I had experienced really disgusting dreams prior to awakening; I could not remember a thing about the dream content but I had a horrible feeling of disgust, hanging all about me. The feeling was so intense that I felt as if I should shower.

I hadn't taken anything into sleep for my body to work on (via a SleepMagic request) so whatever my body had been attempting to bring to my attention, it was something that she had generated on her own. I had the sense that she was trying to get my attention in order for me to give her permission to address whatever it was, so right then and there I set her up with a SleepMagic invocation for that night.

Now … some background: the years 2017 and

2018 were particularly disturbing for me but, precisely because of that, they were also particularly productive from the standpoint of addressing emotions and fears that had been hiding so deep within me that I had not known that they were still disturbing my body at a physical level. Mentally, I was disappointed and angry at the shift that had occurred at the highest political level of the country in which I live. I was aware that I was disappointed and angry but I was not aware, until an unidentified illness kept me bedridden for three weeks, that my body had also been seriously disturbed by the political shift. Almost as soon as I realized that she, too—not just my mind—had been affected, I realized *why* it had affected her. There was a quality of meanness and hatred and greed that permeated everything that the current political administration was doing … and those were exactly the same kinds of energies that had belonged to the many men that had used and abused my body for their own purposes when she was very young.

Because all of these people and all their noxious energies were now permeating the atmosphere, were constantly on the radio, and constantly on the Internet, and because I was both angry and feeling helpless in the face of such an onslaught, she—my body—recognized it. She recognized the same feelings from when we were very, very young … because bodies never forget. My mind could rationalize the feelings away for a while, allowing me to occupy myself with other things, like my painting, which had never been better, but she—my body—couldn't do that. For her, because she had access at a deep and unconscious feeling level to what I was going through, she was reliving the terror of our shared childhood. Here we were again, at the mercy of greedy old men who wanted what they wanted and would get it— because they could—at any cost. She was terrified that the worst was upon us, again.

I'd thought I was pretty well healed from the abuse I'd gone through ... until then. By the end of 2017 I was feeling better, feeling more grounded. I was engaged in doing what I could, utilizing the emotional cellular reprogramming that SleepMagic provides on a regular basis whenever I noticed that I was being triggered by something. I was no longer feeling as helpless as I had ... and she—my body—felt better too. Then, one evening, as my husband was outside working on a shed he was building, the scaffolding beneath him collapsed and he fell to the rocky forest floor, face first. I had heard the collapse and looked out the window to see him stumbling down the hill, toward the house, so bloody that I could barely see his face. He had been taking blood thinners because of a problem with his heart that had come up as the result of an accident two years before. It was dusk. We live in the woods, a forty-five-minute drive from the nearest hospital, and twenty-five minutes from the closest ambulance. I had no choice but to move as quickly and efficiently as I could to collect ice and towels to get him in the car and drive as fast as I could to the hospital.

It was like a nightmare, driving on the dark, winding roads, then melting into an interstate competing with speeding semis and rush-hour traffic as I sped to the emergency ward knowing that there was every chance that my husband might bleed to death right there beside me. Once I was able to get him into the hands of the capable attendants, I collapsed into the waiting room chair where I sat to wait for news. He was determined to be in critical but stable condition and, after some remarkable surgery, he recovered over the next few months, but for me, the incident was the coup de grace for my already struggling body consciousness. It was five months later before I even realized how poorly I was functioning. But other people had noticed. My daughter was concerned that I might be losing my mind. I'd known I "wasn't myself," but I, too, thought I might be slipping into senility, as my mother had not long after I'd confronted her with the memories that had returned to me.

All I knew for sure was that my country seemed to be falling apart. I was falling apart; I couldn't retain a thought in my head for more than a few seconds and I was unbelievably tired. I thought about death a lot ... about how peaceful it would be to no longer be trapped in human form on an insane planet.

I had been creating, for almost the entire year prior to having the aforementioned horrible dream, what had been clearly the best work I'd ever done. I had finally managed to create paintings that allowed both halves of my evenly balanced brain to take part in the work and I was thrilled by the results I was getting. My subject matter was unusual ... and always the same: an image of a single fish hovering over a kind of "quilted" abstract background ... it seemed odd to me at first, but about six months into it I finally realized, from an intellectual standpoint, exactly what it was that I *was* doing: each painting I was creating was a *fish out of water*, all of them creatures out of their element ... and the minute I realized consciously what I had been unconsciously creating was the minute I realized why it felt so right ... and probably the reason why SleepMagic had come to me in the first place so many years before ... it was because of the disconnect between the Spirit aspect of the Self and the Body aspect of the Self. That very disconnect was and is the whole reason that SleepMagic exists: to try to help make peace between these two vastly divergent forms of consciousness by enhancing communication between them!

Then, on the afternoon after the dreadful dream that I previously described, as I was varnishing a recently completed piece, musing on the whole Body/Spirit split, on how being in a body is such a chore ... WHAM! It hit me. My body had been trying to get my attention ...

because I'm an idiot. (Something I've been very conscious of since it was revealed to me—loudly! But with loving humor—in a hypnopompic trance one morning decades ago.) Here I am, in this amazing body, this body that has not just survived two illnesses that kill most of the people who get them, but has even transformed itself, transformed its very cellular structure, in my behalf, and here's me bitching and moaning to myself—and, unintentionally, to my hard-working, dedicated body—for almost two years about wanting to leave her, to go "back into Spirit."

I'm not sure "idiot" is an encompassing enough word to cover my attitude. I was embarrassed of myself. SleepMagic for that night was a really big apology to my body.

But here's the thing: it's a built-in conundrum. Life is hard; life can be mean; life can be violent and ugly and frightening. Ideally, all of that is balanced by the remarkable beauty that life also brings, by experiences that the body itself has, like orgasms, like the ability to enjoy really good food, or cuddling. If the ephemeral spirit does not embody, then Spirit misses the show because embodying is the only way Spirit gets to experience that. But sometimes when the show gets particularly difficult, there is this little niggling desire to desert the premises. I had been guilty of that and, apparently, my body felt it … and she had probably been feeling it for quite some time. That morning—the morning of the disgusting dream— she must have decided that she'd had quite enough of my "poor me" attitude and let me have it by bringing me a dream I couldn't ignore. It made me sad to have let my body down in this way after everything that she has done for me … and it woke me up at every level of my being.

That night I gave her permission to make whatever adjustments she needed to make in order to assist me in aligning more closely with the life that she and I are living together, so that I could better align myself with life itself.

She and I, we are close; we understand each other. But, thanks to her, "I" have a mind and that mind can be a troublesome thing, longing for the impossible, frustrated with things that cannot be changed. I work daily to keep that mind in line. I strive to remain in the Now Moment … but sometimes things march into that Now Moment that remind me all too vividly of aspects of life that I wish I could ignore. But it would be irresponsible of me to simply dismiss those things. I am learning—slowly—how to live with them, how to deal with them … that is all *about* Life, and my body is in life. She has her own existence and I had somehow overlooked that fact and had disrespected her and all that she has done and continues to do for me and on the morning of the dreadful dream, she showed me that so that I might really want to hold up my end of our relationship with considerably more integrity.

What has happened since then is nothing short of remarkable. I have been able to use SleepMagic to assist me in staying more fully present in the Now Moment (which, as an added benefit, helps me to better remember things), to assist me in becoming more acutely aware of when I may be caught up in a wave of melancholy or remorse so that I can allow the feelings to move through me without becoming attached to them. I have been conscious of the fact that I have been following her guidance in the creation of my paintings, that this "best work of my life" is almost entirely attributable to the intelligence of my body. Metaphorically, I've put my mind on a short leash. Oh, it walks off on its own every once in a while, but I catch on far more quickly to its diversions and re-mind it of its real job, which is keeping track of the many various aspects of reality that one needs to keep track of in order to navigate daily life.

The Needs of the Body

One night in the fall of 2018, utilizing SleepMagic, I took a fairly simple request into sleep asking my body for feedback on cutting out an exercise that a physical therapist had recommended—some years ago—that I do "every day." At the time the therapist had recommended the exercise, I'd been driving a lot and was having a relentless pain in my right hip joint—that's my "gas pedal" leg. I'd been doing the exercise she'd prescribed—basically leg lifts—for some years but by 2018 I was no longer driving nearly as much as I had been two years before.

My body gifted me with a pleasant, positive response to my inquiry. She was happy; I could stop the exercises. After fully wakening, I turned to sit on the edge of the bed in order to rise and, as I stood up, there arose from my mind the following enthusiastically presented sentence, "It feels so good to be alive!"

Whoa!

That took me aback.

I mean, yeah, life was good, and, sure, it had been challenging in hundreds of ways, but I'd have been the last one to say that it's anything but a privilege to be able to experience it … still, dang … it was flat out awesome to have my body generate that message for me to hear. (As goofy as I can be, she still loves me; we'd been consciously working together via SleepMagic for almost fifteen years at that point.)

I figured that I must be doing something right and I

was also pretty sure that my body's response to my request had been possible because of the relationship that she and I have established via SleepMagic since, after what was—at that point—fifteen straight years of SleepMagic, I seemed to be more open than ever to her "messages." It's a very different sense of what it is to be alive when you understand that "your" life exists as a cooperative experience with your body and his or her or their life.

I posted the experience on the SleepMagic Facebook page expecting feedback, after all, the past two years in the United States had been anything but pleasant or easy. Why would my body be moved to exclaim, "It feels so good to be alive," at a time when hatred and violence, hypocrisy and meanness were blanketing the globe?

The answer to that is simple: she's a body, an animal body, and like any animal being, if her physical needs are met, she's got everything she needs and we— my body and I—have been fortunate enough, as of this writing, to have been blessed with an existence in which we have what we require to sustain ourselves. In addition to that, we have the pleasure of knowing the physical comfort of a fulfilling intimate relationship with another human being. We are truly content.

The needs of the body are—first—to survive, and then, if possible, to feel good.

Every one of us is a walking conflicting agenda. The body has its needs, its agenda, as has been previously mentioned, but both the Mind and the Spirit also have agendas. This is precisely where we run into trouble. The mind, while really useful in circumstances where control of some sort needs to be exercised, where its skills and its ability to create order can be utilized, can be a bit of a goofball when it confronts things that it cannot possibly control.

The spirit is useful at motivating, at taking chances,

and at attempting to open the mind to trying new things but its urges may well be out of sync with the body's abilities. There is a kind of negotiation going on at all times between the three levels of being but it is the body that always has the appropriate answer because without the body there is no threesome, hence, no human life as we know it since the spirit has no way to express itself on this Earth without a body, and without the body, neither would the mind exist.

Because the mind seems driven to control, SleepMagic becomes exceptionally useful. I have written three books so far on SleepMagic and its use so I won't get into that in great detail here. Suffice it to say that what this particular form of emotional cellular reprogramming allows to happen gives the person utilizing the technique access to information that would otherwise be unavailable because of the mind. The SleepMagic technique allows you to turn over to the intelligence and consciousness of the cells of your body for examination and decision-making questions, conundrums, and situations in which you just don't know where to turn, as well as various solutions that your mind may have come up with in response to those things, so that your body can let you know the proper way to proceed in order to keep you—and your body—alive and well and safe.

In a nutshell, via the SleepMagic technique, you present your body respectfully with an idea that you have or situation that you are struggling with, and you request that your body allow you access to its intelligence on the matter. In this technique, you are using your mind to formulate the words that you will say to your body but it is the body that will generate feeling information that will allow you to know what steps to take next. The challenge is keeping the mind out of the way once those feelings have been generated, allowing the body's feelings to be recognized as important information and—

very specifically—avoiding any mental "interpretation" of those feelings.

The mind will strongly want to interpret things because the mind wants things to make sense ... but feelings don't make sense ... they *are* sense ... or perhaps more correctly, they are sensing. It's convenient though that you can train the mind to keep itself on track. It takes awareness—self-awareness—and some persistence, but it doesn't take all that long. I can't say this for sure, but I have a sense that the reason it doesn't take all that long is that the mind—which tends to go into overdrive and wear itself out—prefers to be at peace. So once it catches on that you're serious, that it *can* be at peace, that it really can "go off-duty" from time to time, that it can step aside and allow the body to take charge more often, it's more than happy to just kick back and devote itself to doing sudoku or rebuilding an engine or writing letters.

The mind is not a monster and mind is not a bully. The mind is simply a good friend that is trying way too hard to help.

Vibration

Now we must address an aspect of the body that has everything to do with everything: vibration. Everything vibrates. As I am writing this, on the day after a vicious winter storm that has literally ripped trees right out of the ground, I am listening to the sounds of a generator outside my office window, a generator that is getting power into this house. Its vibration is rhythmic and unavoidable, in much the same way as the vibration of a jackhammer is rhythmic and unavoidable. But it is not just noisy, huge machines that vibrate; everything vibrates and most vibrations, while rhythmic, go unnoticed because they are so small and so gentle. We can easily hear the vibration of our hearts beating but very few people feel the vibration of the individual cells in their bodies yet literally every cell in your body is vibrating at every moment.

When the cells of the physical body are disturbed or assaulted in some way we are thrown into an imbalance, an imbalance that may be—or may seem to be—mental, but the bottom line is always a cellular bottom line; remember, it is the brain that generates our mental faculties and the brain is a physical, cellular thing. When the cells of the body can be restored to their natural rhythm—their natural vibration—the body and the mind can both be assisted in their healing processes. This is becoming more and more widely known, accepted, and utilized in Europe, where vibrational therapies have been made part of many medical programs.

The vibration of the body affects more than just our mental and physical states of being, it affects our "magnetic" capabilities. This vibration that your body generates is what lies beneath the so-called and much-bandied-about Law of Attraction. Do you know why, on the shelves of the self-help section of every bookstore in America, there are hundreds of books on how to be successful? It's because most of those books are wrong. Most of those books are about using one's mind in order to become successful and, because of that, the formulas in the books don't work, so people keep returning to the bookstore looking for another book that will give them what they *think* they need. The mind, there is no doubt, is a useful tool; the mind is good for reading the book. But without the body on board the mind is no more than a calculator and a recorder of information at best.

If the body is carrying information that tells the human being in question that "success" is toxic, or information that successful people are bad or evil, success will elude that person, no matter what thought-concepts (things like "I am a successful entrepreneur") they may have trained their minds to think. No thought process can override the information that cells are carrying and when that information is negative, there is no thought process that can override it. No matter how focused the thinking, it will not be productive. And don't forget, the brain is an organ that is generated by the body; all the cells that carry all this information about success being toxic are right there in the brain that some would-be successful young entrepreneur is attempting to train to "think successfully." So if human being A is reading a book telling them that they need to think, think, think positive, that they need to think "wealth," to think "riches," the only thing that is happening is a seriously uncomfortable disconnect in the neural pathways that are carrying information that says that wealth and riches are toxic, or that you don't deserve them.

This is something that I personally struggled with for years. The worst of the abuse I endured as a child was at the hands of exceedingly wealthy people and as a result, as a child, I formed a cellular gestalt with a supporting mindset informing me that wealth was evil and through most of my adulthood, I struggled to make a living. I was a good person; I knew that. But my body knew that people with a lot of money were bad people. If I wanted to remain a good person—and I did—as far as I knew, I had to avoid having too much money. So no matter which way I turned, no matter what I tried, for the longest time—until I started clearing at an emotional cellular level—I was always just getting by and the body is not really comfortable with just getting by. The stress of it can actually undermine your health. Ideally, we all have what we need to survive ... and, mind you, having an excess, having far more than you need to just survive, can also cause difficulties for the body because having excess generates a different kind of stress. Too much is just as problematic as too little, just for different reasons.

In addition to being preprogrammed by troublesome relationships with money or by people with money, there's a current highly popularized idea of "success" which is based on accumulating more money than one requires to live comfortably. Countless books have been written on the subject of acquiring millions, if not billions, of dollars. Vibrationally speaking, having more than you need is incorrect. It's excessive. One has only to look at nature and the inherent balance of growing things to understand the correctness and efficiency of living in alignment with one's needs.

Real success in life is having what you need to live and living a good life, which is as simple as being in energetic integrity, and treating others with energetic integrity. The vibration of cells in energetic integrity creates a magnetic field that draws to it what will allow those cells to thrive and grow.

The body is exquisitely designed to resonate with other vibrations, with the vibrations that exist in all living things as well as those that exist in the space/time continuum, the eternal realm of shifting possibilities, and thought and energy fields of all sorts. It is your body's access to vibration that allows it to have the distinction of always having the information that you need.

One very simple—and entertaining—example of vibration can be found in the use of what some people might call fortune-telling cards. Fortune-tellers have been around for as long as people have been cataloguing history and probably longer. Our vibrational resonance affects everything we do, so when we sit with a card reader or we draw cards, it is our cellular vibration that is guiding the process.

As a rule, for as long as such cards have been available to the general public, these cards have been used by "readers." I have been such a reader in this lifetime. I read tarot for people for around thirty years. One can, of course, read one's own cards. The problem with reading one's own cards, however, is obvious as most people are simply unable to get enough distance on themselves—on their minds—to read their own cards objectively.

There is a saying in the world of science, "for every action, there is an equal and opposite reaction." This also holds true in the world of fortune-telling cards and vibration. Every card carries a polarity: this, or its opposite. Common knowledge has it that those polarities only show up when the card is "reversed," or upside down but the fact is that while, yes, the card does carry a different vibration when it shows up upside down, it still also carries polarity; both options are potentially possible.

The reason these types of cards work—especially the ones with some history behind them—is because they, too, carry vibration, the vibration that was put in at the time of the creation of whatever particular images are pictured on the card. Because the people who are "picking" the cards also carry a vibration, they will draw to them what their vibration attracts. The reader, because they are present in the vibration of the seeker, is, for all intents and purposes, channeling the vibration of the seeker. That said, the reader has a vibration as well; it is that vibration that attracted the seeker to that reader in the first place. The end result of any reading depends strongly on the nature of the vibrations between the reader and the seeker and the cards and that dynamic is always something to be considered.

Twice in my life I have had one of my hands grabbed, without my permission ... remember my background of massive abuse, and think about the vibration that *I* was carrying that called out to complete strangers at two different times, to simply reach out, grab me, and read my palm! For reasons I was both too young and too stunned to question at the time, I simply allowed each of these people to do so. My body did what she had learned to do from a childhood of abuse: she/I surrendered. I cannot remember the first reading at all. I was not long out of college at the time, working at a small boutique which I was simultaneously stealing from when I could get away with it; I was standing behind the counter and handling a sales transaction with a woman who, mid-transaction, proceeded to "read my palm" without so much as an announcement that she was about to do so. I don't remember a word she said.

I am aware that my energy field is highly active. I don't know how else to say it. I have been known to screw up the operation of a computer just by being near it, not even doing anything. So I suspect that these two people who decided that I needed their information may have been responding to my random, outgoing energy, which, at that time in my life, I was completely unaware of and certainly unable to control.

The second time it happened was when I was working in a casino in Atlantic City as a cocktail waitress, as a Playboy Bunny to be precise. I was walking the casino floor when a man—an older gentleman—reached out and took one of my hands, which was a very bold move on his part as a person can be thrown out of a Playboy Casino for as little as touching a Bunny let alone grabbing one. He gazed into my hand, and in a kind of dreamlike state announced that I was going to have "three marriages or marriage-like relationships" and then told me that I would live a long life and be very happy in my old age. I was in my first marriage at the time, but it had never been really stable. He was right on the money as it turned out. I am, as I write this, in my third marriage, and happier than I could have ever imagined being.

That's an illustration of what I referred to earlier, that the body has access to the vibrations of the whole life. That man in the casino, as he held my hand, essentially read the vibration of my life. There are some people who have that gift; there are also some people who pretend to … like the woman in the boutique whose information rolled off me like water off a duck's back. She didn't resonate with me and obviously the information she shared didn't resonate with me either.

I stopped reading cards for people in a fortune-telling way, years ago. My personal preference has always been to avoid "fortune-tellers." I like to leave my options open and that includes allowing my mind to be free of expectations—especially ones "implanted" from outside of my own energy field—since expectations carry their own vibrations and, if they've been generated by the mind, as they often are, then they are highly likely to be out of alignment with the pure, base vibration of a body. That said, the use of cards—any kind—can be very helpful in showing you what kind of vibration you may be generating at a given time and if you utilize the information you receive with an open mind and the knowledge that the information is bringing to you all the possibilities that it presents—both supportive and challenging—you may be assisting your body in its decision-making process by "feeding" it additional information that it can use when it responds to the opportunities that present themselves.

Bottom line, we carry a vibration. Other people respond to that vibration. When our vibration is pure and clear and high, we attract people and opportunities of a similar vibration. And because all people are not the same, one person's high vibration may be very different from another's and present very differently in the world. One thing is the same, though, vibration is a very physical thing, generated by the cellular intelligence of the body. The mind has a vibration, yes, but remember, the mind is a spirit energy being hosted by the brain, which is an organ in the physical body, therefore the vibration that comes from the mind is a mixed bag.

All those books in the bookstores on how to succeed, on how to get rich, on how to attract a partner, appeal to the expectation-generating function of the brain, which is generally fueled by all sorts of "advertising," familial, societal, and energetic. Centuries ago, the Greek philosopher Socrates is reputed to have said, "Know thyself." There is no better advice ... but it is not necessarily an easy thing to do because of all the expectations that may have been directed toward you throughout your life, on all the direction that has been given to you since you were young, and by all the hype that current commercialism has generated to make you think that you need this, that, or the other thing, or that you need to look a certain way or act a certain way in order to be accepted into some aspect of society that they have duped you into thinking is where you need to be. That is why I strongly recommend the study of yourself via Evolutionary Astrology, so that you can understand what your own personal baseline is as a human being.

As a human being, as a vibrational creature, you are your own best source of information about yourself; to be specific, your *body* is your best source of information about yourself. In my three previous books (*Sleep Magic: Surrender to Success*; *Feng Shui from the Inside, Out*; and *The Sleeping Phoenix*), I address in great detail the art of SleepMagic and how you can easily determine with assistance from your body what opportunities, people, food, activities, etc., will work *for* you and what will work *against* you.

Your body can also help you with many spur-of-the-moment decisions via what is commonly called muscle testing. Most people who are drawn to a book such as this one most likely know what "muscle testing" is, but just so we're all on the same page, I will describe some different approaches to what is known as muscle testing. Muscle testing is a technique used by many so-called alternative practitioners—which is to say that it is used by people who have been trained to help other people achieve healthy strong bodies through ways that are vibrationally or nature based and are intrinsically aligned with the natural functions of the body. The term "alternative practitioners" is one that has been used to recognize clearly the difference between so-called medical practitioners—a.k.a. doctors—and those practitioners that take a different—and generally less pharmaceutical or surgical—approach to health and to wellness.

Muscle testing is a method that is used in determining the body's response to whatever it is that the practitioner is bringing to the body. That might be an herbal medicine, a supposition about a part of the body, a suggested treatment, anything, really, that is being presented to the body in question as a means to discover how the body can improve its state. Some practitioners like to have a person extend their arm while they press down on it as they ask a question or as the person holds the remedy in question in their opposite hand. Some practitioners will have a person sit down and then they push against their client's leg. If the body part in question remains stable and steady in response to the pushing, the "answer" is in the positive: "Yes, this (whatever-it-is) will work for me" or "is correct for me." If the body part being tested is shaky or unstable or simply gives way, that is read as a negative response; the offering in question will not work for that particular body.

In the case of both questions asked and supplements being held, the body is responding via its vibration to the vibration of the incoming information. Any question asked of you sets up the vibration of an answer within the body; your body responds before your mind does ... because it can; because its life depends on immediate responses to the slightest changes around it. The mind can then—almost without interruption—"interpret" that response. Supplements, too, carry their own vibration to which the body will respond.

At its purest, muscle testing is absolutely accurate. It is able to be accurate because the body does respond with strength when it senses that something is good for it or will work for it. Likewise, when the body senses that something will not work for it, is too costly, or even possibly dangerous for it, it weakens. The difficulty, however, lies in the ego/certainty of the practitioner doing the muscle testing because the strength of the practitioner, sure of his or her "diagnosis," can easily overcome the awkwardly sustained position of an outstretched arm or leg. I have both seen and experienced practitioners quite literally forcing a limb to drop, forcing a "negative" answer in order to validate a claim that something, somewhere was wrong or incorrect and needed "fixing."

The best practitioners of muscle testing use very little force. During the years that I was practicing as a certified practitioner of the technique called Body Talk, I was able to discover easily that it takes very little pressure to feel a body giving way as it releases its negative response to what is being presented to it. There is never any need to be forceful with muscle testing. If you seem to be literally fighting off the person who is muscle testing you, I would recommend that you maintain a healthy skepticism about what is going on.

You can muscle test your own truth easily by yourself through the strength and ability that your body has to maintain balance. There are a number of standing yoga poses that allow you to do this easily and effectively. My suggestion would be, if you are unaware of any standing yoga poses, to do a little research, see what pose looks good/easy for you to maintain, and try the poses out. When you find a pose that you feel confident you can easily balance in, practice a bit until you are confident of your ability to hold that pose and once you reach that point, you will have your own built-in muscle testing tool. All you have to do is bring to mind the question or the issue that you are unsure of—or have someone else present it to you—as you are getting into the pose. If whatever you are asking about is correct for you—for your body—your body will easily take the pose and hold it strong. If it is not correct for you—even if you are a longtime practitioner of yoga—you will sense the weakness in your ability to balance immediately. Either you will be strong (a yes answer) or you will not be as steady as you know you can be (negative answer).

You can use muscle testing to get yes/no answers from your body on almost anything from a relationship to a dietary decision. And I only say "almost anything" because, well, I only know what I know … and, just like everyone else, I don't know what I don't know.

Emotions

Another aspect of the functioning of the body is the biochemical phenomenon we label "emotions." Emotions are one of the greatest challenges to keeping the mind in check. Everybody generates emotions to some degree. In the study of Human Design, human beings are categorized into one of four energy types by virtue of, in a sense, the aspect of the being that moves them ... not what *motivates* the person per se, but what *moves* them to—or supports them in being—*in action*. Most people are moved at a very physical level, a desire of the body to "do something." But for some people this desire to "do something" is colored by and moved to action by virtue—and force—of their emotions. Even though many people use the term "feelings" to describe emotions, emotions are—like Spirit—ephemeral, invisible, inescapable and, perhaps most importantly, powerful. Emotion and Feeling are *not* the same. It might be said that Feeling is more like Sensing in that it is more physically palpable than emotion.

We "feel" all the time. We may feel hungry or tired or moved to do something; all those things are motivated by how our body is physically feeling. The mind, of course, comes into play frequently where feelings are concerned because despite the fact that we may feel tired, we may also have a job to do that requires being done immediately. In order to get the job done, we can override whatever we are feeling—or not, depending.

Emotions, however, cannot be as easily overridden. Sadness, love, anger ... the list is practically endless and contains many variations and levels of intensity. One can pretend to ignore an emotion; one may be able to suppress an emotion to some degree, but one cannot override it. Feelings are *linked* to mental activity and can provide a kind of subjective overview of something that is going on in the body, strongly suggesting that you eat, or lie down, or whatever may be needed for the body at the time. Emotions—which are also born of the physical body and its biochemistry—*power* things. You might say that Feelings make suggestions while Emotions scream at you until you do whatever it is that they feel you need to do.

A feeling can be a mental assessment of an emotion or a physical need. In that regard, the feeling is a somewhat "toned-down" interpretation of an emotion, you might say that a feeling is an attempt brought on by the desires of the Spirit Self via the mind to have some conception of— or better yet, control over—the spontaneous generation of the emotion the body is producing. The process is kind of circular, especially when the mind starts making up reasons for why the emotion is occurring. This is usually where people run into trouble because the mind is of dubious value once it starts steamrolling through the uncharted territory of the emotions.

People who are "driven by" their emotional center may be somewhat less likely than those who are not driven by it to assess the potential effects of the actions they generate. That said, one person who is emotionally driven can affect, by their very presence, everyone around them, activating their emotions. Emotions can be contagious. Some of the very best public speakers may be what is termed, in the system of Human Design, emotionally defined. These people can move an audience because they literally "turn them on." The same thing, of course, can happen in any one-on-one relationship with a person who is emotionally defined and this can sometimes lead to problems in the relationship as the person who moves in and out of this emotionally charged energy field can sometimes act in ways that they might not have otherwise, surprising themselves and leading them to assess themselves afterward as to exactly what happened. Why did they do what they did? Why did they say what they said? Why did the person they were talking with respond to them in the way that they did? Generally, there's nothing to be done about it. What's done is done. Understanding why such a hurtful and/or confusing thing might occur, *knowing* that the person they were dealing with is an emotionally defined person—and being able to accept that—is often the only thing that can get a person past such an event. (Yet another reason to explore Human Design.)

It is precisely these kinds of built-in energetics that can cause two people to "fall in love" despite the fact that they argue frequently. While there may be a very real basis for the love, and that love may feel fabulous, there's also a very real basis for potential conflicts. Yes, people can change, but they cannot change the essential nature of their bodies; all they can do is learn how their bodies want to be in the world and figure out how to manage that. (Yet another area where the Mind comes in very handy.)

[Please note that I used the phrase, "the essential nature of their bodies"; I did not say "what their bodies are." Bodies are—emphatically—not things; "things" do not have life in a way that animal creatures do. Human bodies are male, female, some combination thereof, or possibly asexual. "Things" do not have a gender; your body does ... and some have more than one.

I must sometimes resort to the use of the generic identifier, "it," for simple ease of understanding as the English language does not yet have a term for a trans- or multi-gendered identifier.]

Being in a Body

Your body has emotions; you have feelings. It is the emotion that has to be respected first because it is your body that has it and your body has to come first, always ... well, perhaps not in a math test ... but outside of the realm of exercises that are strictly mental, your body and the way that he or she feels about anything—including taking a math test—is the most important thing for you to pay attention to because your body is the ultimate source, via its gut responses and emotional reactions, of what is good for you, to what will work for you, and to what will keep you healthy and alive. And when I say "you," I am talking about your entire three-part being.

The Spirit Self

> *"We are spirits in the material world ... "* —Sting

... and we really are just that: Spirits in the material world ... only most people, even though they may be aware of that fact, fail to grasp the implications of it.

The human body is an animal thing; what makes the human body very different from an animal body is the consciousness that inhabits a human body. That consciousness is an ephemeral thing. Spirit functions in a very different way, as you might expect, from the way that the body functions. Spirits, for instance, do not have to worry about getting hurt. Anyone who has had a child or been around children knows that the children have to be taught about how to avoid getting hurt, about how to stay what we might call "safe." That is precisely because the Spirit aspect of the child knows no fear and the child's body, which has no experience as yet to inform it of what is dangerous and what is not, also tends to have no fear. This is precisely why we refer to people who seem to have no fear as being "high-spirited." Spirit can—and will, if left to its own devices—do whatever it wants.

That is why childhood is such a difficult time for

most people, both parents and children. Parents want to keep their children safe but they are also generally aware that they do not want to "crush the child's spirit." The wise way to handle the situation would be for the parents to explain Spirit to the child, but in all of my years on Earth I have never heard of that happening though I suspect that it has happened, someplace, at some point in time, because there are some people—not many—who understand this and would have the wisdom required to explain to a child how they work. Some Aboriginal tribes, for instance, show evidence that this kind of early teaching might be a part of their culture.

It's not really a difficult thing to explain, it's just that most people, at this point in time, have not been taught to think in this way. We are, each of us, essentially, working partners in an unagreed-upon collaboration between a physical being and a nonphysical being, each of whom are relying, for their communication with each other, on their troublesome offspring that we call the mind.

Many folks, ignorant of the concept of Spirit existing in this particular context, mistake the workings of the mind for the workings of the Spirit. The mind, though, as you recall, is a function of the brain which, while remarkable in its own right, is—like the body—a physical, animal thing that programs and is programmed— vibrationally, emotionally, mentally, and physically—by every living person—and animal—around it. Because of that, the information that the brain generates about life and living can be less than reliable as all that programming influences the "thinking" of the brain in many different ways.

The brain is excellent for solving intellectual problems, it is good for mathematics and writing and doing research and baking cakes and figuring out how to get home and all sorts of things that have to do with manipulating "givens" in the physical world. The brain is, in a sense, a library where we can find specifics and information that we need. It is also excellent at organizing and following directions, making it useful as a sort of a trainer in the process of teaching yourself how to work with all the various aspects of yourself.

The spirit that inhabits the body, however, receives its information from elsewhere. Where? I have no idea. No one does. Well, some people have ideas, but those ideas are impossible to prove and, while they may function for the person who "thought" them, they are usually of dubious value for others. Religion, as we know it in most cases, has developed around the world, in almost every culture, in order to allow people to become comfortable with the idea of Spirit ... and authority. But most of those religions have placed Spirit outside of the realm of humanity itself when it isn't. In fact, Spirit is the very core of humanity. It is the ineffable life-bringing principle inherent in each and every one of us.

If religion understood that each and every human being is Spirit embodied, a great deal of war might be prevented.

Tribalism is still very much with us, encoded in human DNA for purposes of survival, but it's tricky. We need to band together in order to stay alive in nature, but we also need to allow the genetics of "outsiders" to "freshen up" the DNA in order to stay alive on Earth. So, because tribalism is still with us, and because religions that sanction both tribalism and violence are still with us, humanity continues to involve itself in countless wars and murders.

Certainly, there are people who do religion well, just as there are people who do being human well, but those who are unable to embrace global—possibly universal—thinking may do religion very badly and there are many religions that tend to amplify the worst in people, setting themselves and their beliefs up as a standard that cannot be reached by other people or that other people simply do not resonate with. Because of the lack of recognition that every person is Spirit embodied, tribally oriented people tend to be wary of those who do not look like them or think like them and in some cases, end up determining that these "others" must be eliminated.

Spirit doesn't need to murder. It doesn't need to fight. It's Spirit. And we are ALL SPIRIT; there are no "others." Spirit is ineffable; it's invisible; it's intangible. Spirit "needs" nothing. It doesn't need to live anywhere; it doesn't need food.

Spirit is above and beyond concepts of good and evil, existing only to exist. That Spirit chooses, once in a while, to join up with the human animal body, is evidence of desire to experience what it might be like to be physicalized. There are things that are common to the human life that are not common to the Spirit life, things like pain and death. Bodies die. Bodies die in a variety of ways. By entering a body, Spirit can experience that which it cannot otherwise, in much the same way a human being can experience—via an amusement park or virtual reality of some sort—things which it might not otherwise be able to experience.

You may not consider life on Earth to be something equated with an experience in an amusement park; you may not think this whole "living" thing is fun ... and it often isn't. But fun isn't the reason that Spirit comes here to embody; it is, after all, Spirit, and what Spirit does is *experience*. It is likely that Spirit also learns things by being embodied. But our bodies, which also learn things, unlike Spirit, both experience pain and "translate" their experiences—all their experiences—painful and otherwise—into mental information via the system that most of us refer to as "thinking."

Thinking is not a process of Spirit; for Spirit, things simply *are*. The Spirit Self and the human body have that in common. Thinking is a process and a product of the physical body. But, you might counter, thinking is not a physical thing, and you would be correct; thinking is *not* a physical thing. Thinking *is*, however, the output of a physical thing: the brain. The physical brain is not capable of producing, out of its own physicality, Spirit. Spirit simply is and it resides within us. What the physical brain *does* do is produce energy, a kind of electricity that is configured in such a way as to allow us to interpret what we call reality.

The human brain weaves its concepts of reality based on the information that is carried in the cells of the body. Cells have both memory and intelligence. Your body remembers everything that it has ever seen, heard, smelled, touched, or been touched by. Everything. And, unless some form of intervention takes place, it never forgets those things. Ever.

That is precisely why most "talk therapies" do not, technically speaking, "heal" anyone; what talk therapy does is train the mind to *handle* the offending information that the body is carrying around in a way that allows a person to live a more normal life. That is useful. More useful are the numerous therapies and practices that work directly with cellular consciousness at its own level. Emotional Cellular Reprogramming, EMDR, and SleepMagic are a few of the ways that allow the physical body to release unpleasant and troublesome information so that they—and the person in question—can heal at an emotional level, thus allowing the body to generate appropriately supportive messages about life.

The Spirit Self is rarely in need of healing. And I only say it that way because I always like to leave the door open—wide open—for possibility. After all, it is clear that none of us ever knows everything there is to know. For all I know, the Spirit Self doesn't know everything either. But the Spirit Self for sure cannot experience so many of the things a human body can. It may know about them, but it cannot experience them as its Spirit Self. Every form of existence has its limitations.

It is highly likely that most of us have been raised to rely on our minds. It is also highly likely that whenever our Spirit Self raised its head, that we were cautioned about our behavior because that behavior was likely free of any constraints, like safety, for instance. Because childhood lasts for as many years as it does, and because it takes only seven years for information to be fully imprinted into a human body, most of us enter into our adult life—often marked as the age of twenty-one—with the information we've been given by practically every adult around us that "thinking" should guide our every move and that our bodies exist primarily to serve us and to entertain us.

What we are *not* taught is that we are not, in fact, our bodies. Quite the contrary. The mere fact that death is treated as something utterly dreadful sends a potent message: if the body is gone, so are you. But the fact is that "you" are not gone; *you*'ll be back. We'll all be back. Again, and again and again ... Alternately, every manifestation of us is here, on Earth all the time since time is not, as we tend to think of it, linear. Time is, rather, a continuum and in that regard we are always here.

How it is that I happen to have access to this information:

The abuse that began for me at about age four was overwhelming enough that I "left my body." "I"— that is to say, my Spirit Self—left my body, dove into the Earth, and, via the root systems that I found there, traveled up into whatever tree was closest, hanging out in the branches above, observing what was happening to my body below and communicating with her long distance. At the time, this behavior was so second nature for me that I did not realize it wasn't common; it was how I knew to get through life.

The trees taught me everything that I needed to know about how to deal with the abuse that was going on. They allowed me, in a sense, to experience from above and outside, what was happening inside my body, below. They taught me how to sense what was going on in the body or bodies that were using me so that I could respond in a way that would quicken their responses. In the short term, that had the undesirable effect of making me a rather popular item while, in the long term, it elevated my status in what I would later discover was a ritual group.

Also, in the long term, my leaving my body ended up, in a sense, partially separating my spirit consciousness from its own consciousness. It became something that happened so automatically that I was unaware of it until my second husband noticed that I was "not there" during our sexual play. He asked me where I was going when we were having sex and I told him.

I think my body had been waiting for that precise moment because I answered without hesitation and without thinking, "into the trees," I said. He asked me why I was doing that and I told him that that's what I always did because at the time that's all I knew. In fact, if, in my late thirties, someone had asked me if I left my body when I was having sex, I would've laughed out loud. I'm not even sure that I would have known what they meant. The fact that my husband had chosen just that moment, when we had not yet separated from each other, to ask me that question, was probably the only reason that I was able to mentally connect with what I had done as a child, and with the intelligence of my body, an intelligence that far supersedes the intelligence of the mind. It also added a little information to a curious habit that I had had since I was a child, which was to draw myself as a tree.

I was a Being. I was in a Body. And while those two aspects of myself were functioning well enough, it seemed that they were not communicating with each other. On the one hand, I "escaped" the body in order to see or experience what was happening to the body, but from the outside, in. This was probably helpful for maintaining my sanity, but did my body miss me? Was there some kind of integration between body and being that should have occurred as the result of the abuse and did not? Might this be why the memories that the body had collected were repressed? Might they have been kept in safekeeping for the mind, perhaps? For later, when the mind was able to handle it?

Most books are full of answers; this book is full of questions because we know what we know, but we *don't* know what we don't know. And because our minds are so insistent on knowing, we will often attempt to generate answers simply to allow us to have a "reason." Thinking that we know something relaxes us. Actually knowing something—especially when that something is deeply upsetting, possibly even dangerous—can cause extreme anxiety, and can even cause the body to forbid the conscious mind access to certain types of information, for its own sake. What we don't know we know can often hurt us even more than what we know we know.

Prior to my second marriage I had lived a life of promiscuity. In retrospect, I suppose that I may have been what is commonly called a sex addict. I hated myself for the way that I was but I could not, try as I might, stop my behavior. That behavior cost me the custody of my two children from my first marriage as their father had threatened to "make them hate me" by telling them who I really was and how I had behaved. I determined, for my second marriage, because the cost I had paid to enter into it—the loss of my children—had been so high, that I would, come hell or high water, be faithful to the man I was committing myself to.

I tried.

Being in a Body

But what I discovered was that as long as I was in any way attracting men, I had no control over my ability to say no. In an attempt to stop that from happening—because it was apparent to me that my mind and my desire to be "good" were simply not enough—I began to dress in a very asexual, if not actually somewhat masculine, manner. This confused my second husband but it kept me safe ... or so I thought.

And I suppose that it was because I had gone from being an overtly sexual creature to being an almost completely *a*sexual creature, that my second husband began watching a lot of sexual material on television and made no attempt to disguise his appreciation of the women that came our way. I was unable to control my jealousy. It would have been the end of our marriage except for one thing: a rapidly advancing case of diffuse progressive systemic sclerosis, a disease which crept up on me slowly, from the inside, out, and began to turn every part of me that could be turned into scar tissue into scar tissue.

I was killing myself. It took seven frustrating months to get a correct diagnosis and, once I had gotten the diagnosis, and had read up on the disease, only to discover that it was both fatal and incurable, the process sped up. Eventually, I was told that I could look forward to about six more months of an exceedingly painful life. Throughout my young adulthood I had, more times than I can count, drawn myself as a tree; now, it seemed, I was turning into one.

But, as it turns out, scleroderma (the common term for the disease) actually saved my life. The memories of childhood abuse had been tamped down well below the level of my waking awareness but my Spirit Self, which scleroderma forced me to allow to lead the way, seemed to be set free by the crippling and restriction of the body which it inhabited. It brought me dreams and visions and songs and began to provide me with direction to which I paid attention and against all odds, in a few years' time, the disease left, leaving me a very different person … yet not entirely freed of my past.

Post Script: the original draft for this book was begun in 2018 but the rising political turmoil of 2019 – most specifically the "suicide" of Jeffrey Epstein more than anything else—triggered what I hope is what was left of the horrifying experience of being sexually trafficked as well as having been exposed to the deaths of innocent children. In August 2019, I began what is to be a series of acupuncture treatments, an experiment to see if my fingers and hands, which still remain severely crippled from scleroderma, can be loosened a little. Neither my practitioner nor I have known at any point what to expect … as of this writing, we still don't as we have only just completed the third treatment. That said, we have a little more of an idea since, following the third treatment, which was the first treatment directly on my fingers (the first two treatments had been what she termed "exorcisms," which she felt I needed and I agreed).

Two days following the third treatment I experienced the most horrible dream that I have ever had in my life. I will not describe it here. Suffice it to say that I awoke in a traumatized state, crying, frightened, and thrashing about. My husband held me for close to an hour as my legs pumped, in an attempt to run away from my abusers.

So frightened had I been as a young person, that when our gym class was taken out to run around the track, my legs would cramp up every time. I couldn't do it; I couldn't run. I couldn't afford to run because I knew that if my body was ever allowed to run that she would most likely take to running when she shouldn't and that I would likely be murdered because of it. I knew the dreadful things that had happened to my sister when she tried to avoid serial rapes to which we were subjected and so my approach had been to submit.

I have been afraid to speak of this publicly because I am very well aware—and Jeffrey Epstein was living proof—that the ring of exceptionally wealthy men (and the wives who supported them) are still quite active and as dangerous as they ever were. But my body made it clear to me in September of this year it was time for me to speak publicly—or at least write publicly—about these things, for as long as they are secret, they will continue.

On the morning in September of the horrible dream, as my husband held my body tight, all the repressed childhood desires to run moved through my legs and found an outlet at last, my voice found an outlet too and it cried out, "so many things I'm not supposed to say," over and over again.

I may not be entirely free of my past, but I know now that I am a lot freer than I once was and I am—my body is—living proof of the intelligence and memory of the cellular consciousness of the body.

About the Author

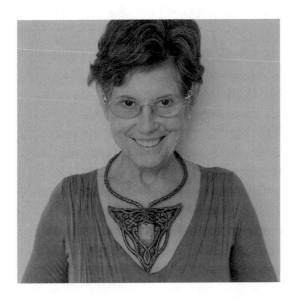

Rev. Victoria Pendragon. D.D., B.F.A. is 1 part Author, 1 part Artist, and 1 part Mentor. She is also a miracle and a medical anomaly, having survied two diseases that are considered to be btoh incurable and fatal. When very young, she experienced what some people would call a Walk-In event which probably served her well in dealing with being sexually trafficked and experiencing incest as a child. These physical assaults on her mind and body led to an early life fraught with an uncontrollable promiscuity and eventually led to the loss of both her children to their birth father.

Acquiring the disease, diffuse progressive systemic sclerosis, which turned her entire body into collagen and crippled her hands, turned her life around. Her approach to life was totally altered and by the time the disease miraculously departed, she was a different person, her body restored to its former softness and her mind opened to a level of consciousness she had not known since she was a child.

During the course of the disease process she had been told by many people but she was a healer but only after two very powerful angelic visits did she embrace that calling and then, wholeheartedly, becoming an ordained InnerFaith minister and taking numerous certifications in various healing modalities.

Today, she lives, very much a hermit, the old hills of Appalachia, drawing, painting, writing, and acting as a mentor for those who feel they need assistance in learning the technique, Sleep Magic, was gifted to her in dream in 2003. This is the happiest and most content she has ever been.

Books by Victoria Pendragon

Born Healers
Published by: Ozark Mountain Publishing

Feng Shui From the Inside, Out
Published by: Ozark Mountain Publishing

Sleep Magic
Published by: Ozark Mountain Publishing

The Sleeping Phoenix
Published by: Ozark Mountain Publishing

Being In A Body
Published by: Ozark Mountain Publishing

**The Grail: A Beginners Guide to Spiritual Realization,
Self-Actualization & Metaphysics**
On 8 CDs, Self-Published

My Three Years as A Tree
Self-Published

The Little Chakra Book
Self-Published

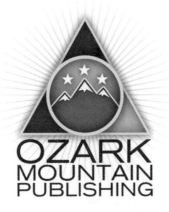

OZARK
MOUNTAIN
PUBLISHING

For more information about any of the above titles, soon to be released titles,
or other items in our catalog, write, phone or visit our website:
Ozark Mountain Publishing, Inc.
PO Box 754, Huntsville, AR 72740
479-738-2348/800-935-0045
www.ozarkmt.com

If you liked this book, you might also like:

A Small Book of Comfort
by Lyn Willmott
Soul Speak
by Julia Cannon
Divine Gifts of Healing
by Cat Baldwin
Little Steps
by James Ream Adams
Judy's Stroy
by L.R. Sumpter
Tales from the Trance
By Jill Thomas
Croton
By Artur Tadevosyan

For more information about any of the above titles, soon to be released titles,
or other items in our catalog, write, phone or visit our website:
Ozark Mountain Publishing, LLC
PO Box 754, Huntsville, AR 72740
479-738-2348
www.ozarkmt.com

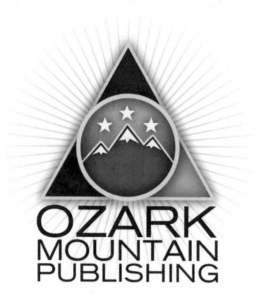

For more information about any of the titles published by Ozark Mountain Publishing, Inc., soon to be released titles, or other items in our catalog, write, phone or visit our website:

Ozark Mountain Publishing, Inc.

PO Box 754

Huntsville, AR 72740

479-738-2348/800-935-0045

www.ozarkmt.com

Other Books by Ozark Mountain Publishing, Inc.

Dolores Cannon
A Soul Remembers Hiroshima
Between Death and Life
Conversations with Nostradamus,
    Volume I, II, III
The Convoluted Universe -Book One,
    Two, Three, Four, Five
The Custodians
Five Lives Remembered
Jesus and the Essenes
Keepers of the Garden
Legacy from the Stars
The Legend of Starcrash
The Search for Hidden Sacred Knowledge
They Walked with Jesus
The Three Waves of Volunteers and the
    New Earth
Aron Abrahamsen
Holiday in Heaven
Out of the Archives – Earth Changes
James Ream Adams
Little Steps
Justine Alessi & M. E. McMillan
Rebirth of the Oracle
Kathryn/Patrick Andries
Naked in Public
Kathryn Andries
The Big Desire
Dream Doctor
Soul Choices: Six Paths to Find Your Life
    Purpose
Soul Choices: Six Paths to Fulfilling
    Relationships
Patrick Andries
Owners Manual for the Mind
Cat Baldwin
Divine Gifts of Healing
Dan Bird
Finding Your Way in the Spiritual Age
Waking Up in the Spiritual Age
Julia Cannon
Soul Speak – The Language of Your Body
Ronald Chapman
Seeing True
Albert Cheung
The Emperor's Stargate
Jack Churchward
Lifting the Veil on the Lost Continent of
    Mu
The Stone Tablets of Mu
Sherri Cortland

Guide Group Fridays
Raising Our Vibrations for the New Age
Spiritual Tool Box
Windows of Opportunity
Patrick De Haan
The Alien Handbook
Paulinne Delcour-Min
Spiritual Gold
Holly Ice
Divine Fire
Joanne DiMaggio
Edgar Cayce and the Unfulfilled Destiny of
Thomas Jefferson Reborn
Anthony DeNino
The Power of Giving and Gratitude
Michael Dennis
Morning Coffee with God
God's Many Mansions
Carolyn Greer Daly
Opening to Fullness of Spirit
Anita Holmes
Twidders
Aaron Hoopes
Reconnecting to the Earth
Victoria Hunt
Kiss the Wind
Patricia Irvine
In Light and In Shade
Kevin Killen
Ghosts and Me
Diane Lewis
From Psychic to Soul
Donna Lynn
From Fear to Love
Maureen McGill
Baby It's You
Maureen McGill & Nola Davis
Live from the Other Side
Curt Melliger
Heaven Here on Earth
Henry Michaelson
And Jesus Said – A Conversation
Dennis Milner
Kosmos
Andy Myers
Not Your Average Angel Book
Guy Needler
Avoiding Karma
Beyond the Source – Book 1, Book 2
The Anne Dialogues

For more information about any of the above titles, soon to be released titles,
or other items in our catalog, write, phone or visit our website:
PO Box 754, Huntsville, AR 72740
479-738-2348/800-935-0045
www.ozarkmt.com

Other Books by Ozark Mountain Publishing, Inc.

The Curators
The History of God
The Origin Speaks
James Nussbaumer
And Then I Knew My Abundance
The Master of Everything
Mastering Your Own Spiritual Freedom
Living Your Dram, Not Someone Else's
Sherry O'Brian
Peaks and Valleys
Riet Okken
The Liberating Power of Emotions
Gabrielle Orr
Akashic Records: One True Love
Let Miracles Happen
Victor Parachin
Sit a Bit
Nikki Pattillo
A Spiritual Evolution
Children of the Stars
Rev. Grant H. Pealer
A Funny Thing Happened on the
    Way to Heaven
Worlds Beyond Death
Victoria Pendragon
Born Healers
Feng Shui from the Inside, Out
Sleep Magic
The Sleeping Phoenix
Being In A Body
Michael Perlin
Fantastic Adventures in Metaphysics
Walter Pullen
Evolution of the Spirit
Debra Rayburn
Let's Get Natural with Herbs
Charmian Redwood
A New Earth Rising
Coming Home to Lemuria
David Rivinus
Always Dreaming
Richard Rowe
Imagining the Unimaginable
Exploring the Divine Library
M. Don Schorn
Elder Gods of Antiquity
Legacy of the Elder Gods
Gardens of the Elder Gods
Reincarnation...Stepping Stones of Life
Garnet Schulhauser

Dance of Eternal Rapture
Dance of Heavenly Bliss
Dancing Forever with Spirit
Dancing on a Stamp
Manuella Stoerzer
Headless Chicken
Annie Stillwater Gray
Education of a Guardian Angel
The Dawn Book
Work of a Guardian Angel
Joys of a Guardian Angel
Blair Styra
Don't Change the Channel
Who Catharted
Natalie Sudman
Application of Impossible Things
L.R. Sumpter
Judy's Story
The Old is New
We Are the Creators
Artur Tradevosyan
Croton
Jim Thomas
Tales from the Trance
Jolene and Jason Tierney
A Quest of Transcendence
Nicholas Vesey
Living the Life-Force
Janie Wells
Embracing the Human Journey
Payment for Passage
Dennis Wheatley/ Maria Wheatley
The Essential Dowsing Guide
Maria Wheatley
Druidic Soul Star Astrology
Jacquelyn Wiersma
The Zodiac Recipe
Sherry Wilde
The Forgotten Promise
Lyn Willmoth
A Small Book of Comfort
Stuart Wilson & Joanna Prentis
Atlantis and the New Consciousness
Beyond Limitations
The Essenes -Children of the Light
The Magdalene Version
Power of the Magdalene
Robert Winterhalter
The Healing Christ

For more information about any of the above titles, soon to be released titles,
or other items in our catalog, write, phone or visit our website:
PO Box 754, Huntsville, AR 72740
479-738-2348/800-935-0045
www.ozarkmt.com